KETOGENIC DIET 101

TABLE OF CONTENTS

INTRODUCTION

Although ketogenic diet has been around for nearly a century, it's speedily gaining quality these days. There is a reason why keto is extremely regarded. It's not a fade diet, it really works, and it is tremendous health advantages additionally to weight loss. Once on the keto diet, you're feeding your body precisely what it wants, whereas eliminating toxins that may slow it down.

The keto diet focuses on low carbohydrates, that the body converts into energy to assist speed up weight loss.

Carbohydrates are converted into glucose and cause a spike in insulin. As the insulin enters the bloodstream to process the glucose, that becomes the most supply of energy. A spike in insulin can also result in storage of fats. The body uses carbohydrates and fats as energy, the former being the primary source. Therefore the additional carbs you consume in your daily diet, the less fat is being burned for energy. Instead, the spike in insulin can lead to additional fat storage.

When you consume fewer carbohydrates, the body goes into a state assigned to as ketosis. Thus, the name for this low-carb diet.

Ketosis helps the body survive on less food. By being in ketosis, you 'train' your body to utilize fats as the main supply of energy in place of carbs, just because there's near to zero carbs to start with. Throughout ketosis, the liver breaks down fats into ketones, that permits the body to use the fat as energy. During a keto diet, we don't starve ourselves of calories, but we have a tendency to starve the body of carbohydrates. This makes weight loss simple and natural.

Later on, you'll learn that the keto diet has several further health advantages besides fat loss.

The keto diet is a straightforward diet, however some individuals do miss beans and breads. It takes a bit of getting used to, starting anything new is challenging after all. However, you'll feel much better, both physically and mentally that you'd be happy to avoid carbs once and for all. And having the ability to eat bacon on a diet will have its rewards!

Chapter 1: What is Ketogenic Diet?

The keto diet is a low or zero carbohydrate diet, however it differs from alternative low-carb diets (such as Paleo) in that it deliberately manipulates the ratios of carbs, fats, and protein to transform fat into the body's primary source of fuel. Our bodies are used to using carbohydrates as fuel. Fats, which is a secondary source of fuel, are rarely tapped on. Meaning the additional fat is stored and keeps adding on the pounds.

The only ways that to scale back fat in an exceedingly 'normal' diet are to consume less fat and workout a lot in order to increase energy expenditure over daily calories intake, that's why most people fail to lose weight on conventional diet.

On the opposite, the ketogenic diet uses fat for fuel, which implies it gets used rather than being stored. So, weight loss becomes simple. Additionally to weight loss, the ketogenic diet is known as the "healing" diet. The shortage of sugar intake has been proven to help and prevent several diseases such as cardiovascular disease, high pressure level pressure, cancers, epilepsy, and plenty of symptoms of aging.

The manipulation of carbs, fats, and protein is crucial in order to get into ketosis. It's a state once the body, deprived of the usual carbohydrates and sugar, is forced to use fat as its primary fuel. Therefore the ratio of fats and protein are considerably higher than carbs in general.

Of course, consuming less carbs also means lowering the amount of insulin in your body. Less insulin equal less glucose and fat storage. That's why the keto diet has been so successful in helping individuals with diabetes. It adjusts the sugar level naturally.

The ratio of carbs, fat, and protein can vary. Many people enable themselves up to fifty grams of carbohydrates a day and still lose weight. On a stricter regime, the carb will be between fifteen and twenty grams daily. The less carbs, the faster the weight loss, however the diet is very flexible.

On the keto diet, you don't count calories. You count carbohydrates and change the intake of carbs vs. fat and protein.

A typical keto diet will get sixty percent of its calories from fat, fifteen to twenty five % of calories from protein, and twenty five percent of calories from carbohydrates. The only limitation on the diet is sugar, which you must avoid.

The ketogenic diet is not a fad. Many scientific studies have shown the advantages and benefits and healing effects of ketosis. Discuss the ketogenic diet with your doctor if you are interested in consuming less sugar, losing weight, or as preventive measures against vulnerable health issues.

Chapter 2 -Benefits of Keto Diet

Although ketogenic diet is popularly called as a 'rapid fat loss diet', it is actually more to this than meets the eye. In fact, weight loss and better levels of energy are only by-products of the keto diet, a form of bonus. It has been scientifically verified and proven that the keto diet has several extra medical benefits

Let's begin by stating that a high carbohydrate diet, with its several processed ingredients and sugars, has absolutely no health benefits. These are merely empty calories, and most processed foods ultimately serve solely to rob your body of the nutrients it has to stay healthy. Here is a list of actual benefits for lowering your carbohydrates and eating fats that convert to energy.

Control of Blood Sugar

Keeping blood sugar at a low level is critical to manage and prevent diabetes. The keto diet has been proven to be extremely effective in preventing diabetes.

Many people suffering from diabetes are also obese. That makes a simple weight-loss regime a natural. However the keto diet does more. Carbohydrates get transformed to sugar, which for diabetics can result in a sugar spike. A diet low in carbohydrates prevents these spikes and permits additional management over blood sugar levels.

Mental Focus

The keto diet relies on protein, fats, and low carbohydrates. As we've mentioned, this forces fat to become the first supply of energy. This is not the normal western diet, which may be quite deficient in nutrients, particularly fatty acids, which are needed for proper brain function.

When people suffer from psychological feature diseases, such as Alzheimer's, the brain isn't using enough glucose, so becomes lacking in energy, and the brain has difficulty acting at a high level. The keto diet provides an extra energy supply for the brain.

A study by the American Diabetes Association found that Type 1 diabetics improved their brain function after consuming coconut- oil.

That same study indicated that individuals who suffer from Alzheimer's may experience improved memory capacity on a keto diet. Those with Alzheimer's have seen improved memory scores that might correlate with the quantity of ketones levels present.

What does this study mean to an average person? With the emphasis on fatty acids, such as omega 3 and omega 6 found in seafood, the Ketogenic diet is likely to fuel the brain with the additional nutrients to help achieve a healthier mental state. The brain tissue is made up largely of fatty acids (you've heard fish referred to as "brain food"), and the increased consumption of those fatty acids will logically lead to improved brain health.

Our body does not produce fatty acids on its own; we can only obtain it through our diet. And the keto diet is rich in fatty acids.

A diet high in carbohydrates will result in a "foggy" brain, where you have difficulty in focusing. Focusing becomes easier with the augmented energy provided by the keto diet. In fact, many people who have no need or desire to lose weight use the keto diet to improve and enhance brain functions

Increased Energy

It's commonplace, and has become almost normal, to feel tired and drained at the end of the day as a result of a poor, carbohydrate- laden diet. Fat is a more efficient source of energy, leaving you feeling additional vitalized than you'd on a "sugar" rush

Acne

While most of the benefits of a keto diet are well-documented, one benefit catches some people by surprise: better skin and less acne. Acne is fairly common. 90% of teens suffer from it, and plenty of adults do, as well.

While it was always thought that acne was at least exacerbated by poor diet, controlled research is still being conducted. However, many people on the keto diet have reported clearer skin. There may be a logical reason. A 1972 study found that high levels of insulin can cause the break out of acne. Since a keto diet keeps insulin at a low and healthy level, it may very well affect skin health.

In addition, acne thrives on inflammation. The ketogenic diet eases and reduces inflammation, therefore enabling the body to decrease acne eruptions. Fatty acids that are found in abundance in fish are a known anti-inflammatory.

While analysis and researches is still being done, it appears likely that a keto diet has beneficial effects for clearer, healthier, more glowing skin.

Keto and Anti-Aging

Many diseases are a natural result of the aging process. Whereas there haven't been studies done on humans, studies on mice have shown neuron improvement on a keto diet.

Several studies have shown a positive effect of the keto diet on patients with Alzheimer's unwellness. What we do know is that a diet filled with good nutrients and antioxidants, low in sugar, high in protein and healthy fats, whereas low in carbohydrates, enhances our overall health. It protects us from the toxins of a poor diet.

There is also research indicating that the exploitation of fatty acids for fuel rather than sugar may decrease the aging process, probably because of the negative effects that sugar has on our overall wellbeing.

In addition, the straightforward act of eating fewer and consuming less calories is a matter of basic health, because it prevents obesity and its implicit side effects.

Until there, studies have been restricted. But, taking in consideration the powerful positive effects of the keto diet on our health, it is logical to assume this diet will facilitate the process of growth in a more natural way while delaying the natural effect of aging. A standard western diet laden with sugars and processed foods are definitely detrimental to heading off the signs of aging.

Keto and Hunger

Hunger is one of the key reasons why diets fail. People who diet feel hungry and deprived and simply surrender. A low carbohydrate diet naturally leaves people feeling full and satisfied. Less hungry means people will truly persist on the diet longer while consuming fewer calories.

Keto and Eyesight

Diabetics are conscious that high blood sugar can cause a higher risk of developing cataracts. Since the keto diet controls sugar levels, it will facilitate retain eyesight and help prevent cataracts. This has been shown and proven in several studies involving diabetic patients.

Keto and Autism

We know the keto diet affects brain functions. In a study on autism, it was found that it also has a positive effect on autism. Thirty autistic children were placed on the keto diet. All showed improved in autistic attitude, especially those on the milder autistic spectrum. While more studies are needed, the results were extremely positive.

Chapter 3 – Keto Diet and Cancer

Cancer has changed into a serious disease in our modern society. Whereas cancer was not an outsized issue before the 20th century (it did exist, of course), our modern diet and inactive lifestyle have made cancer the second primary reason behind death, with 1600 American dying from this disease every day. It seems that our bodies do not react well to being exposed to daily toxins.

While any cancer treatment should be guided by your doctors, itis a good idea to discuss the ketogenic diet and what it can do to help in the treatment of this disease.

A cancer-specific ketogenic diet may consist of as much as 90 percent fat. There is a really smart for that. What doctors do grasp is that cancer cells feed off carbohydrates and sugar. This is what helps them grow and multiply in number.

As we have seen, the ketogenic diet dramatically reduces our carbohydrate and sugar consumption as our metabolism is altered. What the ketogenic diet does, in essence, is take away the "food" on which cancer cells feed and starves them. The result is that cancer cells may die, multiply at a slower rate, or decrease.

Another reason why a ketogenic diet is able to hamp the expansion of cancer cells is that by reducing calories, cancer cells have less energy to develop and grow in the first place. Insulin also helps cells grow. Since the ketogenic diet lowers insulin level, it slows down the growth of tumorous cells.

When on the ketogenic diet, the body produces ketones. Whereas the body is fueled by ketones, cancerous cells are not. Therefore, a state of ketosis may facilitate reducing the size and growth of cancer cells.

One study monitored the expansion of tumors in patients suffering from cancer of the digestive tract. Of those patients who received a high carbohydrate diet, tumors showed a 32.2 percent in growth. Patients on a ketogenic diet showed a 24.3 percent growth in their tumor. The difference is quite significant.

Another study concerned five patients who combined chemotherapy with a ketogenic diet. Three of these patient went into remission. Two patients saw a progression of the disease when they went off the ketogenic diet.

More studies are needed, but these numbers are hopeful.

The ketogenic diet may facilitate preventing cancer from occurring in diabetic patients in the first place. People with diabetes have a higher risk level to develop cancer because of elevated blood sugar levels. Since the ketogenic diet is extremely effective at lessening the levels of blood sugar, it may prevent the initial onset of cancer.

From what research has discovered so far, ketogenic diet may:

1. Stop the expansion of cancer cells.

2. Replace cancerous cells with healthy cells.

3. Change the body's metabolism and enable the body to "starve" cancer cells by depriving them of needed nutrition.

4. By lowering the body's insulin level, the ketogenic body may prevent the onset of cancer cells.

On a keto diet specifically for cancer, your fats ought to75 to 90 percent, protein 15-20 percent, and fewer than 5 percent carbohydrates.

Foods to Eat

1. Egg, including yolks

2. All green, leafy vegetables, as well as cauliflower, avocado, mushrooms, peppers, cucumbers, and tomatoes.

3. When choosing dairy, choose full-fat version of **cheeses,** butter, sour cream, yogurt, and milk.

4. Eat nuts like walnuts, almonds, filberts, and sunflower and pumpkin seeds.

Foods to Eat in Moderation

1. Have one serving of root vegetables, such as yams, parsnip, carrots, and turnips per day.

2. Fruits contain sugar, so treat them like candy. One small piece per day.

3. A glass of dry wine, vodka, whiskey and brandy once a week. No cocktails with sugars.

4. A small piece of chocolate with 75 percent or higher cocoa content once a week.

Foods to Avoid

1. Any food containing sugar, including cereals; soft drinks, juices, and sports drinks, candies, and chocolate. Limit artificial sweeteners as much as possible.

2. Starchy food like pasta and potatoes, breads, potato chips, and French-fries, cooking oils, and margarine.

3. All beers.

Chapter 4 – Keto Diet and Epilepsy

The initial use of the ketogenic diet had nothing to do with weight loss or diabetes management, for which it is now so well-known. Instead, the diet was created by a doctor in 1924 to help his patients suffering from epilepsy (brain disease.).

Epilepsy is a nervous system disorder that can bring on recurrent seizures at any time. The symptoms can be spasms and convulsions, or an unusual psychological view of the world. In any case, it is caused by abnormal brain activity. The severity of the symptoms varies from person to person. A person is diagnosed with epilepsy only if he or she suffers from more than two seizures in one full day. Anyone can suffer from this disorder, however it looks to affect young children the most, maybe because the young brain is still in a state of development.

Seizures are often managed by drugs. Sometimes they work; sometimes, they don't.

As far back as 1924, however, Dr. Russell Wilder of the Mayo Clinic conducted groundbreaking research and created the keto diet to help children suffering from brain disease. It absolutely was effective, but doctors lost interest when new anti-seizure medications came on the market. It was easier for them to prescribe medication than to discuss diet.

However, people who used the ketogenic diet to treat seizures continued seeing good results and outstanding success.

Today, doctors are returning to using the low carbohydrate, high-fat diet to treat their patients. The results have been extremely promising.

In 1998, the Journal of Pediatrics published a study involving 150 children who experienced seizures despite taking popular anti- seizure medications. The kids were placed on the keto diet for one year which the researchers assessed their progress.

Eighty-three percent of the subjects were still in the study after 3 months. Over one-third of the kids showed a 90 % decrease in seizures. At the end of the year, slightly more than half of the subjects had remained on the diet, and a quarter of them experienced a 90 percent decrease in seizures. The numbers indicate that the ketogenic diet has a tremendously positive effect on children who suffer from seizures. The researchers consider it more effective and practical than medication in several cases.

For anyone with children who experience seizures, the inclusion of a ketogenic diet in the child's treatment should be discussed with his or her doctor (physician).

Another research on the effects of the ketogenic diet on childhood epilepsy involved 145 children. The children were separated into 2 groups, with one group being treated with medication whereas the second group receiving a ketogenic diet. Seventy-four percent of the ketogenic diet group were successful in reducing seizures.

There have been more studies of childhood epilepsy and the ketogenic diet. These have sparked new and considerable interest within the medical profession.

Chapter 5 – Keto Diet and Pressure

One-third of American adults suffer from high blood pressure. It is a significant health problem that can lead to heart attacks and strokes. It is clear that the higher the blood pressure, the greater the risk. Aging and fatness greatly increase the possibilities of developing high blood pressure.

Blood pressure is generally treated with a variety of medications, some of which can have side effects. The best blood pressure is 120/80. High blood pressure is the result of hypertension, and the causes aren't always clear, however we live in an increasingly tense world, and more and more people are dealing with high blood pressure.

It is a known fact that individuals suffering from high blood pressure frequently carry excess belly fat and can become at risk for type 2 diabetes. To get at the origin of all these problems may require a change in lifestyle.

The symptoms of high blood pressure can be caused by an overload of carbohydrates in the diet, more than the body is able to handle. As we've discussed, carbohydrates are converted into sugars, which boost the body's blood sugar level, forcing the body to produce additional insulin. Insulin stores fat, and an excess of insulin can lead to fatness. All of this can have a negative effect on your blood pressure.

Consuming fewer carbohydrates decreases both the level of insulin and the blood pressure level. This easy dietary change can make a huge difference in your blood pressure.

In an important study released in the Archives of Internal Medicine, 146 overweight people took part in a weight-loss experiment. The people were divided into two groups. The first group was put on a keto diet containing a maximum of 20 grams of carbohydrates, whereas the second group was given the weight-loss drug orlistat, additionally to being counseled to follow a low-fat regimen.

Both groups showed similar weight loss. What amazed the researchers was that half of the keto group showed a reduction in blood pressure, while only 21 percent of the low-fat diet group had any decrease in blood pressure. While weight loss itself would bring about a lowering of blood pressure, the study suggests that a decrease in carbohydrate intake can help lower blood pressure even more.

It was found that potassium specifically had a huge effect on lower hypertension. Doctors recommend at least 4,700 mg of potassium each day for anyone wishing to lower his or her blood pressure.

Foods high in potassium are:

- Avocado
- Acorn squash
- Bananas
- Coconut water
- Dried apricots
- Pomegranate
- Salmon
- Spinach
- Sweet potato
- White beans

While all these foods are allowed on the ketogenic diet, limit your intake of sweet potato and beans, which are starchy and can contain a high level of carbohydrates.

Chapter 6 – WHAT DO I EAT ON A Keto Diet?

Some people associate the ketogenic diet with the bad word "fat," and are fast to dismiss it. Nothing could be further from the reality. Fat is allowed, because it is converted into energy. Our body needs healthy fats to thrive. Other foods on the diet could not be healthier. When you're eating keto, you're filling your body with nutrition. Let's take a look at the foods you'll be eating.

As this book has already noticed, the elimination of processed foods and sugar is one of the effective and best things you can do for your health in general. Processed foods are filled with toxic preservatives that do nothing for you but rob you of your good health. Fresh is always better. Once buying something at the market, get into the habit of reading labels. They can be very sneaky and revealing.

Keep your carbohydrates below 50 grams a day, and you'll feel the difference. A stricter keto diet will contain approximately 20 grams of carbohydrates a day.

Food to Eat on a Ketogenic Diet

1. Seafood:

Everyone knows about the healthy fatty acids, vitamins and minerals in seafood. Only a few people eat enough. The ketogenic diet encourages the consumption of all things from the sea. Shrimp and crabs are carb-free, and other shellfish contain only a low amount of carbohydrates.

Fatty fish, like salmon and sardines, are extremely suggested due to their high omega-fatty acid content. Fish truly is brain food. Enjoy at least two servings or more of seafood a week on the ketogenic diet. Simple canned tuna counts as seafood.

2. Vegetables:

Can a diet that recommends unlimited green, leafy vegetables be anything but healthy? They are extremely low in carbs and bursting with vitamins, antioxidants, and the fiber we need daily. Green vegetables such as broccoli, spinach, and kale are believed to reduce the risk of heart diseases and cancer.

Cauliflower and turnips can be prepared to look and taste like rice or mashed potatoes, with much less starch and carbohydrates.

"Starchy" vegetables, such as potatoes or beets do have carbs and should be limited on the ketogenic diet.

3. Dairy Foods:

- There are cheeses to satisfy everyone's taste. They are high in fat content for energy, high in protein and calcium, and low in carbohydrates.

- Yogurt and cottage cheese are a great source of protein and calcium. They are low-carb and fit well into the keto lifestyle.

- Be sure to stick with plain yogurt, as the flavored types contain a lot of sugar, as are the so-called "low fat" versions of yogurt. You can flavor yogurt and cottage cheese yourself with a few berries and nuts.

4. Avocados:

Avocados are truly "superfood." They are high in important vitamins and minerals, including potassium. According to a study, avocados are also believed to help lower cholesterol by 22 %.

Loaded with nutrients and delicious taste, avocados only have 2 grams of net carbohydrates. Use them in salads and sandwiches.

5. Meat and Poultry:

The ketogenic diet lets you eat plenty of meat. Meat contains very few carbs and is full of protein to help you build muscles. Whenever possible, choose healthy, grass-fed meats, which are higher in fatty acids.

6. Eggs:

Eggs are high in protein and contain a mere 1 gram of carbohydrates. As they are also cheap, they are ideal for everybody on a keto diet.

Eggs also make you feel full, thereby helping you eat less. Many people take pride in only consuming the whites of eggs, but the true nutrition lies in the yolk, so be sure to eat the egg in its entirety.

7. Coconut Oil

Too many people are unfamiliar with coconut oil, another "superfood." It is perfect for people dealing with diabetes and has been used with Alzheimer patients.

Coconut oil can be used in most recipes in place of butter or oil. You can also use it for frying and sautéing.

8. Dark Chocolate

Did you know that dark chocolate has a high amount of antioxidants? As a matter of fact, dark chocolate is reaching superfood status. Chocolate with 80 % or higher real cocoa powder can decrease your blood pressure.

An ounce of 80% dark chocolate contains 10 grams of carbs, so it definitely counts as a healthy snack. Remember the lower of cocoa content, the less healthy the chocolate will be. Milk chocolate does not count as a healthy chocolate.

Foods to Avoid on a Ketogenic Diet

The ketogenic diet has a lot less restricted foods than many other diets. Sugar, of course, must be avoided. That doesn't mean you can't enjoy your snack or sweet desserts. There are many keto-friendly recipes that substitute unsweetened apple sauce for sugar in baked goods. Substitute sweeteners like Stevia can also be used in moderation.

Keep in mind that fruits are healthful, but they do contain a great deal of sugar, so limit the amount you eat to just a few slices a day. Fruit juices are concentrates that have vitamins but lack fiber. And their sugar content is extremely high. Read the label on any bottle of juice before buying. The best juices are "green" with just a hint of fruit for flavoring.

Be careful with cereals. Most are packed with sugar and robbed of any nutrients. Many claim, "nutrition added," but all that means is that all nutrition has been removed and replaced with a small amount, and a whole lot of sugar for taste. 100% bran cereal will fit into your ketogenic diet, and you can sweeten it with a handful of berries. Just pay attention to examine all labels in the cereal aisle. They can be very tricky. Also, keep in mind that honey, too, is considered as sugar.

Totally omit white starches from your diet. They are nothing but empty calories. This includes white bread, pasta, and rice. Buy the wholegrain version, instead, and enjoy in moderation.

Legumes and beans are healthy for you, however they are high in carbs. You can have them occasionally; just make sure you keep it within your daily 20 – 5o carb-gram count.

Alcohols tend to be empty calories, but certain spirits will be better for you than others. Beer is filled with carbs and should be off your ketogenic diet. The expression "beer belly" exists for a reason. Enjoy a glass of wine, instead. Of course, there are variances in different types wine. Dry wines contain a minimum amount of sugar, while sweet dessert wines contain much more.

Pure alcohol such as whiskey and vodka are carb-free, but they do contain calories, so have a care. Mixing alcohol for fancy cocktails usually creates a haven for sugar, so avoid those.

Wine coolers may be a tasty treat, but in reality, they are just sugary sodas with some added alcohol. They should definitely not be on your ketogenic diet at any time.

Chapter 7 –Keto Diet for rapide weight loss

Many individuals mix up the keto diet with low carb diets or paleo diets. However, there are considerable differences of which you should be aware.

Keto v. Low Carb

A low-carb diet can be anything it wants to be, as long as it is low in carbs. And "low" is rarely defined. On a low-carb diet, you simply make random food choices that slow down your carb intake randomly. Since there is no real number, you might still be consuming too many carbs.

Most importantly, what the low-carb diet lacks is that all-critical ketogenic state that turns carbohydrates into fats and provides your body with a new and effective source of fuel. This can leave you very hungry and tired.

The ketogenic diet has a specific ratio of carbohydrates to fats to protein. This manipulation is critical, and it's why a low carb diet won't work as well, if at all.

Keto v. Paleo

The Paleo is also a low-carb-type diet. It is based on the assumption that eating the way our cavemen ancestors did, i.e., meat and no carbsohydrates, sugars, or grains, is the healthiest type of diet.

There are problems with this reasoning. First, our ancestors never experienced the kind of illness that we face. The keto diet is specifically a "healing" diet that is meant to benefit the body in many ways and help prevent diseases. The paleo diet doesn't do that.

Also, the paleo diet is based on eating meat rather than manipulating the ratio of fats, carbs, and protein to achieve a ketogenic state that uses fat as fuel.

Ketogenic Diet

Basically, ketogenic is low-carb, but it is much more.

There is a reason the ketogenic diet has become so popular. It helps improve your overall wellbeing in addition to helping you lose weight. You have more energy throughout the day, and you feel sated and full, thereby reducing the cravings for unhealthy snacks. In essence, you are eating less, but better. That's what makes the ketogenic diet so unique and successful.

The keto diet is not magic pill created by some gurus. Countless studies and testimonials are able to back the effectiveness of this diet. It is a scientifically proven method that balances your body's fat intake to help achieve optimal weight loss.

By using fat instead of sugar as your primary source of energy, the keto diet induces a state of ketosis, which is achieved when your body stops receiving carbohydrates to turn in glucose. The fewer carbohydrates you consume, the more you force your body to burn fat for energy instead of storing it.

This is why it is possible to lose weight so quickly on the keto diet. It counts carbohydrates instead of calories. Using fats as an additional energy source is what ketosis is all about. It is a natural state that helped our hunter-gatherer ancestors survive in early days.

They feasted on low-carb foods when they could, and fasted when food was scarce. Fat was stored and converted into energy during the scarce times. The ketogenic state is a natural human state, which makes the ketogenic diet so powerful and successful. In addition to the benefits of the keto diet, most people simply enjoy the way it makes them feel better.

Weight loss results on the keto diet differ among individuals, depending on their specific body composition. But weight loss has been the consistent result of people who've been on the ketogenic diet. The ketogenic diet is known as the best weight-loss diet, as well as the healthiest.

A 2017 study divided Crossfit-training subjects into two groups, with both groups following the physical training, but only one group combined the keto diet with the training. The results indicated that those on the keto diet decreased their fat mass and weight far more than the other group.

The keto diet group showed an average of 3.5 kilo weight loss, 2.6 percent of body fat, and 2.83 kilos in fat mass, while the other group lost no weight, body fat or fat mass. Both groups showed similar athletic performance ability.

A 2012 study splitted overweight children and adolescents into two group; one was put on a ketogenic diet, the other on a low-calorie diet. As in other ketogenic studies, the children on the keto diet decreased their weight, fat mass, and lowered their insulin levels clearly more than the low-calorie group.

Besides more quick weight loss, a decided advantage of the ketogenic diet over a low-calorie diet is that people actually stick to the keto diet. A low-calorie diet will help you lose weight, but you may be constantly feeling hungry and deprived. That is the main reason most diets fail. Hunger and deprivation are not a part of the ketogenic lifestyle.

Ketosis Explained

As we have stated previously, the keto diet isn't magic. It is proven and well-tested science. Ketosis is a natural occurrence that happens when you don't feed your body enough carbs and it is forced to look for energy elsewhere.

You have undoubtedly experienced ketosis when you've missed a meal or have exhausted your body with rigorous exercise. Whenever these things happen, your body helps you out by raising its level of ketones. But, most people eat enough sugar and carbohydrates to keep ketosis from happening.

We love our sugar and carbs, no matter how bad they are for us, and our bodies will happily use them as fuel. And since our bodies want to help us out, it turns any excess glucose into fat and stores it for future use. Stored fat translated into those ridiculous belly fat that you never want.

The more you restrict your carbs consumption, the more your body will produce ketones. It really has no other options. When we reduce the amount of carbs that we eat, our body will still provide us with energy, however it must turn to another source. And that alternate source is fat that was so thoughtfully stored for emergencies. The result is a state of ketosis. It happens when our body breaks down the fat into fatty acids and glycerol.

Researchers have discovered most of what they know about ketosis from people who fast, thus depriving them of all sources of energy. After two days of fasting, the body is starting to produce ketones as it breaks down the available protein and begins to use stored fat for fuel. Ketosis is the natural process the body goes through when deprived of other sources of energy.

Clearly, going on a keto diet is healthier than fasting. Ketogenic should become a lifestyle, not a fast weight-loss method. The main reason it is so beneficial is that ketones offer protection against illness and damages that can affect the body. As mentioned before, ketogenic diet is an excellent tool to prevent many diseases and preserve health and strength longer.

Planning your keto meals will depend mostly on your goals. Are you trying to lose weight, or are you on the keto diet to alleviate the symptoms of some disease? The average ketogenic diet will consist of 4 meals per day, with a total of 100 grams of protein, 25-50 grams of carbs, and 140-160 grams of fat. This can certainly be adjusted to your personal needs.

For example, if you are on a ketogenic diet to improve cognitive functions, you may want to increase your fat intake to 90 grams a day for optimal results.

Benefits of Intermittent Fasting on Keto

The science behind the ketogenic diet is that the body burns fat when deprived of other sources of fuel. Intermittent fasting is a deliberate deprivation of food and takes the concept a step further. We're not talking long-term fasting.

Intermittent fasting while on a ketogenic diet meant having 2 meals a day or fasting for one day a week. The fasting time gives the body a chance to rest and rid itself of toxins. It provides an extra boost to the weight-loss benefits of ketogenic and is a great way to jump-start the diet. For weight loss, the ketogenic diet, combined with intermittent fasting, will help you achieve your goal faster and easier.

Chapter 8 - Getting Started on the Keto Diet

You're ready for a new and improved you. Congratulations. There are so many wonderful benefits to the keto diet, you can expect many positive changes, both physical and mental. So, let's not retard and get the journey begin.

Clear Your Pantry

We're sure you have plenty of willpower, but there is no need to confront a kitchen full with tempting sugars and carbs.

Make a clean sweep and pack the offending items in a box. Then donate the loot to a needy neighbor or a soup kitchen. They will value your gesture, and you are on your way to a ketogenic lifestyle. If you have family, try to get them engaged. If they refuse to refrain from eating carbs and sugar, at least insist they do so away from home. It's a fair request.

Weigh Yourself

The ketogenic diet does not require you to live by the tyranny of the scale. As a matter of fact, as you build up healthy muscles, you might notice a slight initial gain. That's great, so don't be afraid.

You must, however, have an idea of what your beginning point is. If you opted for the ketogenic diet only to lose weight, you will be able to track your progress. But don't become a slave to the scale. The occasional weigh-in, maybe once a week, is enough.

What about Your Favorite Meals?

Perhaps the very thought of surrender your favorite foods has prevented you from getting started on the ketogenic way of life. Relax. The truth is, for every dish that you love and can't live without (yes that includes cheesecake and mashed potatoes!), you can easily find a low-carb substitute that is just as tasty.

First, let's consider items at your market labeled "low carbs." Labels are frustratingly deceiving, and you'd have to be a nutritional expert to understand them. All-too-frequently, off-the-shelf low carbohydrates products have simply replaced sugar for carbs, so don't fall for that bit of deceit. You need to learn to read labels with the diligence that you'd read your wealthy uncle's will, however your best bet is to stay away from these products and simply find healthier substitutes. The same goes for anything labeled "low fat," which inevitably means added sugars.

Craving a taco? Use a lettuce wrap rather than a taco shell. Do you want rice or mashed potatoes? Grate or rice a cauliflower, and you will not be able to tell the difference. Can't give up your favorite pasta dish? Turn a zucchini into "zoodles" by cutting it like slices or using a spiral cutter and enjoy your pasta. You absolutely have to have your favorite dessert? On the keto diet, you can. Just bake with almond flour and use unsweetened applesauce and/or avocado to create some sweet smoothness.

Learn about coconut oil, which can be used as a butter substitute in sautéing, frying, and baking. Coconut oil has incredible health benefits, especially for Type-2 diabetics.

On the ketogenic diet, you'll be able to enjoy all your favorite meals in better way.

Always Stay Hydrated

The ketogenic diet tends to decrease your insulin level, so your kidneys may be excreting more liquid than usual. Be sure to drink plenty of water.

Condiments Can Be the Enemy

Don't assume condiments don't count on a diet. On the ketogenic diet, they most certainly do. Ketchup is filled with sugar. Not all salad dressings are equal. Read the label, and never opt for the "fat-free" version. They have merely substituted sugar for fat.

Ordering salads when eating out is one of your best options, but be aware of the dressing that the restaurant serves. Either ask about the ingredients, or better, bring your own salad dressing. Don't hesitate to do that, even in a posh eatery where the Maître d' might become spastic at the sight of you pulling salad dressing out of your bag.

Keep Track of Your Ketone Level

It's very important to remain aware of how your body is responding to the ketogenic diet at the beginning of the diet. You can do so by doing a simple urine test. You can also purchase a blood ketone meter. It is highly recommended to perform the test early in the morning.

Friends and Family Can Be Annoying – Bless Their Hearts

Those nearest and dearest to you may not often understand what you are doing. When eating as a group, they may put subtle pressure on you to "just try a bite," or "one slice of cake won't kill you." Or worse, "but I cooked it especially for you!"

It will take resolve to stick to your diet. It may help to fill up on keto-friendly snacks before you sit down and eat. Enjoy some nuts, an avocado, or just a leg of chicken before you eat, and you will be less tempted.

Celebrate!

Celebratory occasions, especially if you're the guest of honor, can be a huge obstacle. When the gang at the office or your parents enter a room with a cake yelling "Surprise!" on your birthday, it's hard to refuse. So, try being a bit sneaky, instead.

By all means gush over the offering. You are expected to do that. You can even help cut slices. Then, discover a sudden and irresistible urge for coffee, which you verbalize loudly and clearly. Gently remove yourself from the center of activity to get coffee for yourself and anyone else. By the time anyone notices, hopefully they have missed the fact that you haven't eaten anything.

Traveling

Traveling while on the ketogenic diet can be a challenge, so be well prepared. Pack a personal blender with some avocados and bananas for a few quick and healthful smoothies. Pack some anchovies or tuna for protein.

Eating Out

Eating out isn't as difficult as you may think. Even fast-food places have salads, these days. In any restaurant, stick to meat and vegetables and forego the potatoes and noodles.

You can even navigate the tricky maze in a Chinese restaurant. While abstaining from rice, you can enjoy the following: clear soups, steamed fish with vegetables, egg foo young, stir-fried dishes, Mu Shu without the wrappers are just a few suggestions. Ask your server if your meal can be prepared without cornstarch which is usually used as a thickener.

Even if you end up in a fast food place that doesn't have salad, simply toss the buns from your burger and just eat the meat. You can do the same at a friend's house or at a BBQ.

Exercise

The ketogenic diet will build muscle mass and give you added energy. Don't forget to integrate exercise into your daily routine. It can be as simple as walking more, taking the stairs, or joining a gym.

How Long Should You Stay on a Ketogenic Diet?

The amount of time spent on the diet can vary and must be discussed with your doctor. Many people who use the ketogenic diet for weight loss remain on the diet for several weeks, until they have achieved a goal, then they turn to a paleo diet or other maintenance eating. You do not want to lose weight only to return to your old eating habits.

If you are on the ketogenic diet for medical or therapeutic reasons, check with your doctor to ascertain if you should remain on the diet for a longer period of time.

Chapter 9 – Keto Recipe

You can take your favorite recipes and turned them "keto." Here is a few recipes to show you how easy it is. It might be an excellent idea to buy a ketogenic cookbook for your kitchen.

Two of the most important ketogenic recipes are the simple cauliflower rice and "zoodles." They couldn't be easier to prepare. People can get frustrated on the ketogenic diet when they ask for pasta and rice. These two recipes definitely satisfy those cravings; they taste just like the real thing. The zoodles can be used for any pasta dish.

Invest in a calorie counter, as you will need it.

Omelet Muffins

Make plenty of these ahead of time. They'll go fast.

Ingredients:

1 tbsp. butter

10 eggs

Salt and pepper to taste

½ cup diced ham

¼ cup drained spinach

¼ cup diced onion

¼ cup chopped red bell pepper

¼ cup shredded Pepper Jack cheese

Directions:

Preheat the oven to 350 degrees.

Coat a muffin pan with non-stick spray.

Whisk the eggs, then stir in the remaining ingredients. Fill the muffin pan with the mixture

Bake for 25 minutes.

Nutritional Facts: Calories 155; carb. 2 g; fat 10 g; protein 12.5

Breakfast Casserole

This is a delicious casserole everyone can enjoy. It will leave you satisfied until lunch.

Ingredients:

10 eggs

¼ cup whipping cream

1 cup ricotta cheese

1 diced onion

Salt and pepper to taste

1 package thawed frozen spinach

1 cup sliced mushrooms

1 lb. crumbled sausage meat

Directions:

Preheat oven to 350 degrees.

Whisk the eggs, whipping cream, ricotta cheese and onion well Season with salt and pepper.

Add the spinach, mushrooms, and crumbled sausage.

Bake for 30 minutes

Keto Pancakes

Serve these pancakes with butter and sugar-free syrup or with berries.

Ingredients:

1 ¼ cup almond flour

2 tbsp. honey

1 ¼ cup almond flour 2 tbsp. honey

Dash of salt

1 tsp. baking powder 1 tsp. cinnamon

6 beaten eggs

¼ cup plain Greek yogurt 3 tbsp. melted butter

1 tsp. lemon extract

Directions:

Stir the flour, baking powder, and cinnamon in a bowl.

Combine the eggs, honey, yogurt, lemon extract and butter in another bowl. Slowly stir the egg mixture into the flour mixture.

Use two tablespoons of batter and drop on a hot griddle. Cook for 4 minutes, then flip and cook for another 2 minutes. Continue until all batter has been used.

Nutritional Information: 413 calories; 34g fat; 18.4g carbohydrates; 16.3 g protein.

Apple Red Cabbage

Cabbage is a great vegetable to have on keto. This red cabbage side dish is yummy.

Ingredients:

8 slices of bacon, cut into pieces

1 large diced onion

1 peeled and sliced apple

2 cup chicken broth

3 tbsp. red cider vinegar

2 tbsp. coconut palm sugar or sugar substitute, such as Splenda

1 tsp. ground cloves

½ tsp. allspice

½ tsp. nutmeg

Salt and pepper to taste 1 shredded red cabbage

Directions:

Fry the bacon in a skillet until crispy. Add the onion and saute for 5-6 minutes.

Stir in the broth, sugar, vinegar, spices, salt and pepper. Add the cabbage and cook on low for 45 minutes.

Nutrition Facts:160 calories; 7.8 g fat; 16 g carbohydrates; 4 g protein.

Cinnamon Granola

Store-bought granola usually has a high sugar content.
Try this instead.

Ingredients:

1 cup chopped walnuts

½ cup shredded coconuts

¼ cup sliced almonds

2 tbsp. sunflower seeds

½ tsp. cinnamon

1 tbsp. coconut palm sugar

1 tbsp. melted butter

Directions:

Preheat the oven to 375 degrees.

Combine the walnuts, shredded coconut, sliced almonds, and sunflower seeds. Add cinnamon and coconut palm sugar and stir into the nut mixture.

Spread the mixture in a single layer on a baking sheet. Drizzle with the melted butter.

Bake for 20 minutes.

Nutrition Facts: 180 calories; 19 g fat; 4.1 g carbohydrates; 4 g protein.

Herbed Omelet with Smoked Salmon

You can enjoy this omelet anytime, but a breakfast of protein and fatty acids gets the day started right.

Ingredients:

2 tbsp. butter

2 beaten eggs

1 tsp. tarragon

1 tsp. thyme

Salt and pepper to taste

1 tbsp. butter

2 tbsp. chopped onions

4 very thin tomato slices

2 smoked salmon sliced

1 tsp. capers

Directions:

Whisk the eggs and add the tarragon, thyme, salt, and pepper. Melt the butter in a skillet and add the beaten eggs and chopped onions.

Cook for 3-4 minutes, until the eggs begin to set.

Transfer the omelet to a plate and top with the tomato and salmon slices. Sprinkle with capers. Nutrition Facts: Calories: 239; fat 15 g; carbohydrates 4 g; protein 22 g.

Cheeseburger Salad

This is your favorite cheeseburger without the bun.

Ingredients:

1 lb. ground beef

Salt and pepper to taste

3 cups chopped lettuce

1 small diced onion

1 sliced tomato

¼ cup shredded cheddar cheese

4 tbsp. oil and vinegar dressing

Directions:

Fry the ground beef in a skillet for 4 minutes. Add the onion and cook for another 5 minutes.

Place the beef and onions in a bowl and add the remaining ingredients, except the dressing.

Coat with the salad dressing.

Nutrition Facts: Calories 290; Fat 14 g; Carbohydrates 6; Protein 25 g.

Cauliflower Rice

This very simple recipe is for basic rice. You can dress it up with vegetables, spices, or stir fry it. Use this anytime you need rice as a side dish or in a recipe.

Ingredients:

1 cauliflower head

Directions:

Chop the cauliflower into florets.

Place the florets in a food processor and pulse until you have a rice- like consistency.

Cook the rice in a pan of salted water for 5 minutes.

Nutritional Facts: Calories 21; Carbohydrates 5; Fat 0; Protein 0

Zoodles

These zoodles made from zucchini taste like noodles. A spiralizer is the easiest way to create zoodles, but you can also use a mandolin. Zoodles get soggy very easily, so do not cook for more than 1 minute. Season with butter or shredded cheese.

Ingredients:

1   Zucchini

Directions:

Use a spiralizer to create pasta strands.

Bring a pot of salted water to boil and cook the zoodles for 1 minute.

Bacon-Wrapped Chicken

A very decadent and delicious way to enjoy chicken.

Ingredients:

l bs. Boneless and skinless chicken breast

2 cups chopped spinach

1 cup sliced mushrooms

1 cup cream cheese

½ cup cottage cheese

Salt and pepper to taste

12 slices bacon

Directions:

Preheat the oven to 375 degrees

Combine the spinach, mushroom, cream cheese and cottage cheese in a bowl.

Season the mixture with salt and pepper.

Use a mallet to flatten the chicken pieces to a 1/2 -inch thickness. Use a sharp knife to cut pockets in one end.

Spoon the mixture into the pockets.

Wrap two bacon slices around each chicken piece.

Brown the wrapped chicken in a skillet 5 minutes each side. Place the chicken pieces in a baking dish.

Bake the chicken for 45 minutes. The bacon should be crispy and the chicken done.

Nutrition Facts: Calories 390; Fat 22 g; Carbs 3.9 g; Protein 41 g.

Cobb Salad

This salad is very high in protein. Enjoy.

Ingredients for Dressing:

1 tbsp. olive oil

1 tbsp. white vinegar

1 tsp. Dijon mustard

2 tbsp. diced onion

Salt and pepper to taste

Ingredients for Cobb Salad:

¾ cup cubed cooked chicken

½ cup diced tomatoes

½ cup blue cheese

2 tablespoons blue cheese

1 sliced hard-boiled egg

2 cups chopped greens

1 sliced avocado

4 cooked and sliced bacon slices

Directions:

Arrange the greens on a plate

Arrange rows of chicken, diced tomatoes, blue cheese, egg slices, avocado slices and bacon pieces on top of the greens.

Combine all dressing ingredients. Drizzle the dressing over the salad.

Nutrition facts: Calories 295; Fat 11 g; Carbs 4 g; Protein 22 g

Slow Cooker Pot Roast

This pot roast is prepared without potatoes or carrots. If you add them, adjust the carbs accordingly.

Ingredients:

2 lb. chuck roast

Salt and pepper to taste

1 tbsp. olive oil

2 minced garlic cloves

1 chopped onion

2 ½ cup beef broth

½ cup dry red wine

Directions:

Season the roast with salt and pepper. Salt and pepper the roast.

Heat the olive oil in a skillet and brown the roast on all sides. Place the roast and remaining ingredients in the slow cooker. Stir the ingredients to combine.

Cook on low for 6 hours.

Nutrition facts: Calories 242; Fat 12 g; Carbs 9.8 g; Protein 21g

Spinach and Sausage Soup

This soup is loaded with flavor while remaining very low in carbs.

Ingredients:

1 lb. spicy crumbled Italian sausage 1 tbsp. olive oil

1 chopped onion

2 sliced carrots

1 minced garlic clove

2 tbsp. red wine vinegar

½ tsp. oregano Dash of hot sauce

4 cups chicken broth

½ cup whipping cream

2 cups baby spinach

Salt and pepper to taste

Directions:

Heat the olive oil in a skillet and saute the crumbled sausage for 5 minutes, until it is no longer pink.

Transfer the sausage to a plate and drain on a paper towel. Saute the onion, garlic, and carrot in the same pan.

Deglaze the pan with the red wine vinegar.

Add the chicken stock, whipping cream, oregano and hot sauce and stir well. Season with salt and pepper.

Simmer the soup for 5 minutes.

Transfer the sausage back into the pan and stir in the spinach. Cook for 1 minute to allow the spinach to wilt.

Nutrition facts: Calories 137; Fat 7.8 g; Carbs 2 g; Protein 11g.

Tandoori Chicken

Tandoori chicken is all about the spice marinade. Serve it with some cauliflower rice.

Ingredients:

2 lbs. chicken thighs

Ingredients for Marinade:

1 cup plain yogurt

2 tsp. Lemon juice

Salt and pepper to taste

2 tbsp. olive oil

2 minced garlic cloves

1 tsp. chili powder

1 tsp. grated fresh ginger

1 tsp. garam masala

½ tsp. cumin

Directions:

With a sharp knife, cut several slits into the chicken thighs. Season the chicken with salt and pepper and drizzle with the lemon juice.

Combine the remaining ingredients in a large bowl. Place the chicken in the bowl and coat thoroughly.

Refrigerate up to 24 hours. The longer you marinate, the more flavor is absorbed.

Preheat the oven to 375 degrees.

Line a baking sheet with aluminum foil and layer the chicken on top.

Bake for about 45 – 50 minutes, until the skin is nice and crispy. Nutrition facts: Calories 145; Fat 5.8 g; Carbs 2.3 g; Protein 17g.

Curried Lamb

Filled with exotic spices, this curry dish is perfect with keto rice.

Ingredients:

2 lbs. lamb meat

1 tbsp. olive oil

1 diced onion

3 minced garlic cloves

½ tsp. grated ginger

½ to. Turmeric

½ tsp. curry powder

½ tsp. garam masala

2 cups beef stock

1 cup plain Greek yogurt

1 tsp. lemon juice

Directions:

Cut the lamb meat into small pieces

Sauté the onion in the olive oil for 5 minutes, then add the garlic, ginger, turmeric, curry powder and garam masala. Stir for another 5 minutes.

Add the meat and brown it for 10 minutes.

Pour in the beef stock and simmer for 40 minutes.

Remove from heat and stir in the yogurt and lemon juice. Nutrition Facts: Calories 329; Fat 17 g; Carbs 9.1 g; Protein 36 g.

Cheddar Biscuits

These tasty biscuits are great anytime. They freeze well, so keep them handy.

Ingredients:

2 cups almond flour

1 cup shredded cheddar cheese

1 cup coconut oil

1 cup cream cheese

3 eggs

2 tsp. baking powder

1 tsp. baking soda Dash of salt

Directions:

Preheat oven to 325 degrees.

Cover a baking sheet with aluminum foil.

Place the flour and the cheese in a food processor and pulse to a grainy consistency.

Add the baking powder and baking soda.

Heat the cream cheese and coconut oil in a small pan and warm until they melt. Stir to a creamy smoothness.

Whisk the eggs and add the salt.

Stir the flour mixture into the egg mixture and stir until a dough forms.

Use a tablespoon to drop the dough onto the baking sheet. Bake for 25 minutes. Allow the biscuits to cool for slicing.

Nutrition Facts: Calories 106; Fat 11.1 g; Carbs 2 g; Protein 3.9 g.

Conclusion

Congratulations. You've mastered the keto diet. You've lost weight, feel better, look gorgeous and enjoy the abundance of energy. You've put a lot of effort into improving your health, so what happens when you've achieved your goal and it's time to abandon the ketogenic diet?

It's a hard fact that maintaining your weight loss can actually be more difficult than losing that weight in the first place. Returning to your old and bad eating habits may be all-too tempting. In addition, when you stop the ketogenic diet, your metabolism is likely to slow down, making weight maintenance more difficult.

You certainly don't want to lose momentum and return to the unhealthy, all-American, sugar and carbs swamp, with your lost weight returning. The options below are surely best at maintaining your current state of health.

Consider your options before you stop the ketogenic diet. Have a plan in place and execute it. Since the ketogenic diet provides you with many options, it will be easier to adjust to a maintenance style.

Continue Keto

Continue on the ketogenic diet that has been successful for you, but consume more food. Not different, high-carb foods, but the same foods you ate on the diet, in somewhat larger quantities. You'll be eating more calories.

This will allow you to eat more protein and fats, but keep the carbs level low. This can be a miss process; simply add more calories to your diet and see how your body reacts and adjust accordingly.

This option guarantee that carbohydrates are no longer running your life, as you won't suffer from the cravings you might have had when you begin the ketogenic diet.

Shift from Losing Weight to Gaining Muscles

With the increasing energy you enjoy on the ketogenic diet, you may wish to focus on improving your muscle tone. Many athletes are fans of the ketogenic diet. This means retaining your low body fat but adding muscle and definition. Strong muscles help strengthen bone density and keep you strong as you age.

The best way to gain strong muscles is to consume more calories in the form of lean proteins. This option is difficult to maintain unless to include a resistance training exercise program.

Remain on Low Carb but not on Keto

When you use the ketogenic diet to lose weight, your carbohydrate restrictions are fairly strict. You can still preserve your weight with a low carb diet, but not as rigid as ketogenic. There are many healthy beans and legumes you can enjoy by adding a few more carbohydrates to your diet.

How much more carbs is very personal, because everybody is different. Add a few cups of beans, lentils, or another serving of carrots to your diet each week and see how your body reacts. If you continue to maintain your goal weight, you're on the right track. Add 10 grams of carbs a week until you are satisfied with the results.

The advantage of this option is that it allows you to eat good, healthy foods that were off limits on the keto diet. Having a greater variety of foods from which to choose will make it easier to maintain your weight.

If you find yourself gaining weight, simply cut down on the added carbs just a bit.

Use Intermittent Fasting

Intermittent fasting gives you additional options. Remember that fasting forces your body to burn fat.

Here are some ways you can fast intermittently:

1. Eat what you want for 5 days, then fast for 2 days.

2. Eat two meals a day instead of three, providing for a longer period where you are not consuming food.

When you begin to embrace ketogenic, you will be enjoying all the benefits of healthy eating. By continuing to consume fewer carbs as a lifestyle, your body will remain smooth and strong.

You will also be providing it with ammunition to ward off many chronic illness.